Table of Contents

Reducing Kidney Stone Risk

Resources

Smoothie Recipes

Snack Recipes

Tips

Uncategorized

Vegetarian

Introduction

Kidney stones are usually found in the kidneys or in the ureter, the tube that connects the kidneys to your bladder.

They can be extremely painful, and can lead to kidney infections or the kidney not working properly if left untreated.

What is kidney stone ?

Kidney stones (also called renal calculi, nephrolithiasis or urolithiasis) are hard deposits made of minerals and salts that form inside your kidneys.

Diet, excess body weight, some medical conditions, and certain supplements and medications are among the many causes of kidney stones. Kidney stones can affect any part of your urinary tract — from your kidneys to your bladder. Often, stones form when the

urine becomes concentrated, allowing minerals to crystallize and stick together.

Passing kidney stones can be quite painful, but the stones usually cause no permanent damage if they're recognized in a timely fashion. Depending on your situation, you may need nothing more than to take pain medication and drink lots of water to pass a kidney stone. In other instances — for example, if stones become lodged in the urinary tract, are associated with a urinary infection or cause complications — surgery may be needed.

Symptoms of kidney stones

You may not notice if you have small kidney stones. You'll usually pee them out without any discomfort.

Larger kidney stones can cause several symptoms, including:

pain in the side of your tummy (abdomen)

severe pain that comes and goes

feeling sick or vomiting

When to get urgent medical help

You should contact a GP or NHS 111 immediately if:

you're in severe pain

you have a high temperature

you have an episode of shivering or shaking

you have blood in your urine

What causes kidney stones?

Waste products in the blood can occasionally form crystals that collect inside the kidneys.

Over time, the crystals may build up to form a hard stone-like lump.

This is more likely to happen if you:

do not drink enough fluids

are taking some types of medication

have a medical condition that raises the levels of

certain substances in your urine

After a kidney stone has formed, your body will try

to pass it out when you pee.

Treating and preventing kidney stones

Most kidney stones are small enough to be passed in

your pee, and it may be possible to treat the

symptoms at home with medication.

you have a high temperature

you have an episode of shivering or shaking

you have blood in your urine

What causes kidney stones?

Waste products in the blood can occasionally form crystals that collect inside the kidneys.

Over time, the crystals may build up to form a hard stone-like lump.

This is more likely to happen if you:

do not drink enough fluids

are taking some types of medication

have a medical condition that raises the levels of

certain substances in your urine

After a kidney stone has formed, your body will try

to pass it out when you pee.

Treating and preventing kidney stones

Most kidney stones are small enough to be passed in

your pee, and it may be possible to treat the

symptoms at home with medication.

Larger stones may need to be broken up or removed with surgery.

It's estimated up to half of all people who have had kidney stones will experience them again within the following 5 years.

To avoid getting kidney stones, make sure you drink plenty of water every day so you do not become dehydrated.

It's very important to keep your urine pale in colour to prevent waste products forming into kidney stones.

The kidneys

The kidneys are 2 bean-shaped organs that are roughly 10cm (4 inches) in length.

They're located towards the back of the abdomen on either side of the spine.

The kidneys remove waste products from the blood. The clean blood is then transferred back into the body and the waste products are passed out of the body when you pee.

Very small kidney stones are unlikely to cause many symptoms. They may even go undetected and pass out painlessly when you pee.

Larger kidney stones can cause symptoms, including:

pain in the side of your tummy (abdomen) or groin – men may have pain in their testicles

a high temperature

feeling sweaty

severe pain that comes and goes

feeling sick or vomiting

blood in your urine

urine infection

Blocked ureter and kidney infection

A kidney stone that blocks the ureter, the tube that connects your kidney to your bladder, can cause a kidney infection.

This is because waste products are unable to pass the blockage, which may cause a build-up of bacteria.

The symptoms of a kidney infection are similar to symptoms of kidney stones, but may also include:

a high temperature

chills and shivering

feeling very weak or tired

cloudy and bad-smelling urine

Your GP will usually be able to diagnose kidney stones from your symptoms and medical history.

It'll be particularly easy if you have had kidney stones before.

You may be given tests, including:

urine tests to check for infections and pieces of stones

an examination of any stones that you pass in your pee

blood tests to check that your kidneys are working properly and also check the levels of substances that could cause kidney stones, such as calcium

You may be told what equipment you'll need to collect a kidney stone. Having a kidney stone to analyse will make a diagnosis easier, and may help your GP determine which treatment method will be of most benefit to you.

If you're in severe pain

If you have severe pain that could be caused by kidney stones, your GP should refer you to hospital for an urgent scan:

adults should be offered a CT scan

pregnant women should be offered an ultrasound scan

children and younge people under 16 should be offered an ultrasound – if the ultrasound does not find anything, a low-dose non-contrast CT scan may be considered

TREATMENT

Most kidney stones are small enough to be passed out in your pee and can probably be treated at home.

Treating small kidney stones

Small kidney stones may cause pain until you pass them, which usually takes 1 or 2 days.

A GP may recommend a non-steroidal anti-inflammatory drug (NSAIDs) to help with pain.

To ease your symptoms, a GP might also recommend:

drinking plenty of fluids throughout the day

anti-sickness medicine

alpha-blockers (medicines to help stones pass)

You might be advised to drink up to 3 litres (5.2 pints) of fluid throughout the day, every day, until the stones have cleared.

To help your stones pass:

drink water, but drinks like tea and coffee also count

add fresh lemon juice to your water

avoid fizzy drinks

do not eat too much salt

Make sure you're drinking enough fluid. If your pee is dark, it means you're not drinking enough. Your pee should be pale in colour.

You may be advised to continue drinking this much fluid to prevent new stones forming.

If your kidney stones are causing severe pain, your GP may send you to hospital for tests and treatment.

Treating large kidney stones

If your kidney stones are too big to be passed naturally, they're usually removed by surgery.

Surgery for treating kidney stones

The main types of surgery for removing kidney stones are:

shockwave lithotripsy (SWL)

ureteroscopy

percutaneous nephrolithotomy (PCNL)

Your type of surgery will depend on the size and location of your stones.

Shock wave lithotripsy (SWL)

SWL involves using ultrasound (high-frequency sound waves) to pinpoint where a kidney stone is.

Ultrasound shock waves are then sent to the stone from a machine to break it into smaller pieces so it can be passed in your urine.

SWL can be an uncomfortable form of treatment, so it's usually carried out after giving painkilling medication.

You may need more than 1 session of SWL to successfully treat your kidney stones.

Ureteroscopy

Ureteroscopy involves passing a long, thin telescope called a ureteroscope through the tube urine passes through on its way out of the body (the urethra) and into your bladder.

It's then passed up into your ureter, which connects your bladder to your kidney.

The surgeon may either try to gently remove the stone using another instrument, or they may use laser energy to break it up into small pieces so it can be passed naturally in your urine.

Ureteroscopy is carried out under general anaesthetic, where you're asleep.

Percutaneous nephrolithotomy (PCNL)

PCNL involves using a thin telescopic instrument called a nephroscope.

A small cut (incision) is made in your back and the nephroscope is passed through it and into your kidney.

The stone is either pulled out or broken into smaller pieces using a laser or pneumatic energy.

PCNL is always carried out under general anaesthetic.

Complications of treatment

Complications can occur after the treatment of large kidney stones.

Your surgeon should explain these to you before you have the procedure.

Possible complications will depend on the type of treatment you have and the size and position of your stones.

Complications could include:

sepsis, an infection that spreads through the blood, causing symptoms throughout the whole body a blocked ureter caused by stone fragments (the ureter is the tube that attaches the kidney to the bladder)

an injury to the ureter

a urinary tract infection (UTI)

bleeding during surgery

pain

The best way to prevent kidney stones is to make sure you drink plenty of water each day to avoid becoming dehydrated.

To prevent stones returning, you should aim to drink up to 3 litres (5.2 pints) of fluid throughout the day, every day.

You're advised to:

drink water, but drinks like tea and coffee also count

add fresh lemon juice to your water

avoid fizzy drinks

do not eat too much salt

Keeping your urine clear helps to stop waste products getting too concentrated and forming stones.

You can tell how diluted your urine is by looking at its colour. The darker your urine is, the more concentrated it is.

Your urine is usually a dark yellow colour in the morning because it contains a build-up of waste products that your body's produced overnight.

Drinks like tea, coffee and fruit juice can count towards your fluid intake, but water is the healthiest option and is best for preventing kidney stones developing.

You should also make sure you drink more when it's hot or when you're exercising to replace fluids lost through sweating.

Find out more about preventing dehydration

Depending on the type of stones you have, your doctor may advise you to cut down on certain types of food.

But do not make any changes to your diet without speaking to your doctor first.

The Kidney Stone Diet

Calcium

The US population eats too little calcium for ideal bone health. Because of idiopathic hypercalciuria and probably other factors not as well established, stone formers have an abnormally high risk of bone mineral loss and fractures. So adequate diet calcium is especially important, above 1000 mg per day or more.

Most kidney stones contain calcium oxalate, and oxalate absorption is reduced by high calcium intake. The powerful effect of high diet calcium to lower urine oxalate and prevent calcium oxalate kidney stones is seen in the one diet based stone prevention trial.

Sodium

Because urine calcium tracks with sodium, lowering diet sodium below the US "tolerable upper limit" of 100 mEq (2300 mg) per day, ideally below 65 mEq (1500 mg) per day, can prevent high diet calcium from increasing urine calcium and stone risk. In fact, the combination of low diet sodium with high diet calcium was the only one that produced positive bone mineral balance among menopausal women.

Reduced diet sodium is especially valuable for stone formers. It helps lower blood pressure and they have a higher than normal frequency of hypertension.

Sugar

Refined sugar is a world menace. One half of the molecule is fructose, metabolized directly to fat and capable of inducing insulin resistance in healthy people over as little as 8 weeks. After a dose of sugar, fructose or glucose, urine calcium rises and volume falls, so stone risk rises – all this within a hour or so. Your chocolate bar in mid afternoon is risky! Nationally, sugar is a main cause of obesity and diabetes. Stone formers need to limit it, and so does everyone else. I have – as best I can.

Protein

Skilled scientists have debated if protein excess reduces bone mineral, but all agree it raises urine calcium. Not the commonplace 0.8-1 gm per kg body weight per day recommended for all US people, but values much above that range.

Potassium

Food potassium parallels food anions that when metabolized produce alkali. Good for bones, alkali also signals kidneys to release filtered citrate into the urine where it inhibits formation and growth of stone crystals. Low urine citrate is a recognized stone risk, and before adding potassium citrate supplements one should certainly bring diet potassium up to the US recommendations in hopes that will remedy at least part of the deficit, leaving less for expensive and unpleasant capsules of potassium citrate powder. We generally eat much less than the recommended 120 mEq (4700 mg) per day of diet potassium.

Oxalate

Even high calcium diet will not protect calcium oxalate stone formers against excessive oxalate intakes, so moderation is very important. This site has massive oxalate lists, and our article on low oxalate diet is perhaps the most popular of the over 100 articles here. I have inveighed against a compulsive search for every mg of oxalate in food. It overly constrains diet choices. But diet oxalate matters a lot when stones are calcium oxalate and 24 hour urine oxalate is high enough to convey risk of stone despite that diet calcium has been raised to the US normal range. For this reason, recipes for stone formers need to address oxalate excess.

Kidney Stone Diet Safe Meal Replacement Bar

YIELD: 4 Servings 1x

INGREDIENTS

SCALE1x2x3x

1 Teaspoon vanilla

12 Pistachio nuts

Lilly's butterscotch chips

1/8 Cup Canned Pumpkin

1/2 Cup Peanut Butter

1/2 Teaspoon Pumpkin Pie Spice

56 Grams Egg white protein powder

1/8 Cup Walden Farms sugar free Pancake syrup

Cook Mode Prevent your screen from going dark

INSTRUCTIONS

Mix all ingredients together in a bowl.

Refrigerate for 2 hours, may even freeze if still sticky.

NUTRITION

Calories: 309

Sugar: 4g

Sodium: 169mg

Fat: 21g

Saturated Fat: 4g

Unsaturated Fat: 15g

Trans Fat: 0g

Carbohydrates: 13g

Fiber: 3g

Protein: 20g

Cholesterol: 1mg

Copycat Fiber One Muffins

PREP TIME: 10 Minutes

COOK TIME: 20 Minutes

TOTAL TIME: 30 minutes

YIELD: 12 Servings 1x

INGREDIENTS

SCALE1x2x3x

1/2 Teaspoon vanilla

1 Egg

1.5 Cup Fiber One cereal

1/2 Cup Swerve brown sugar

1/4 Olive oil

1 1/3 Cup of Fairlife ultra milk

Scoop vanilla protein powder

1 Cup Bob red mill high fiber oat bran cereal

2 teaspoon baking powder

Cook Mode Prevent your screen from going dark

INSTRUCTIONS

Preheat oven to 400.

Spray the muffin pan with cooking spray so the muffins don't stick.

Crush cereal in a baggie with a rolling pin or use a glass like I did. Whatever you have available to crush cereal into a finer consistency.

Add milk and vanilla to the cereal and let sit for 5 minutes.

In another bowl, beat egg and add in oil.

Add the rest of the ingredients (baking powder, protein powder, oat bran, and Swerve brown sugar) to the beaten egg and oil mixture.

Add egg mixture to cereal mixture.

Fill the muffin pan.

Place in oven and bake for 20 minutes. Check at 15 with a toothpick; if it comes out clean, they are done. If not, bake for an additional 5 minutes.

NUTRITION

Calories: 114

Sugar: 1g

Sodium: 108mg

Fat: 6g

Saturated Fat: 1g

Unsaturated Fat: 4g

Trans Fat: 0g

Carbohydrates: 23g

Fiber: 5g

Protein: 5g

Cholesterol: 14mg

Banana French Toast with Peanut Butter Maple Drizzle

PREP TIME: 5 Minutes

COOK TIME: 5 Minutes

TOTAL TIME: 10 minutes

YIELD: 1 Serving 1x

INGREDIENTS

SCALE1x2x3x

1 small banana

1 teaspoon cinnamon

2 Tablespoon powdered peanut butter

1 pat of butter

Ezekiel bread

1/4 cup of skim milk

1 whole egg

1 Tablespoon sugar-free maple syrup

Cook Mode Prevent your screen from going dark

INSTRUCTIONS

French toast batter.

Mix together milk, egg, and cinnamon.

Heat a nonstick skillet with a pat of butter.

Drench the bread in the batter.

When the skillet is hot, put in french toast and cook on each side until brown. About 2 minutes each.

While making french toast, make your PB drizzle by following the directions on the PB2 jar. I added more water so that the drizzle could, well, drizzle!When both pieces of toast are nice and brown, put them on the plate and pour on the maple syrup and PB drizzle. Garnish with fruit.

Oxalate: ~38mg Added Sugar: 2g Calcium: 203mg

NUTRITION

Calories: 470

Sugar: 29g

Sodium: 193mg

Fat: 11g

Saturated Fat: 4g

Unsaturated Fat: 4g

Trans Fat: 0g

Carbohydrates: 7

Flourless Banana Pancakes

A flourless, no-added-sugar banana pancake recipe that satisfies that sweet craving.

INGREDIENTS

SCALE1x2x3x

1 ripe banana

2 large eggs

2 tablespoon ground flax meal

1/4 teaspoon vanilla

1 tablespoon coconut oil

Cook Mode Prevent your screen from going dark

INSTRUCTIONS

Mix banana and eggs together in a bowl until smooth.
Add ground flaxseed and vanilla extract; mix the
batter well.

Heat coconut oil in a small skillet over medium-low
heat. Scoop batter, about 1/4 cup per pancake, onto
the skillet and cook until the center starts to bubble,
about 30 seconds. Flip pancakes and cook until
bottoms are lightly browned, 1 to 2 minutes more. I
actually like mine browner than light, but you do you!

NOTES

Oxalate: Less than 5mg   Calcium: 37mg   Added Sugar: 0g   Servings: 2

NUTRITION

Calories: 204

Sugar: 7g

Sodium: 62mg

Fat: 13g

Saturated Fat: 8g

Trans Fat: 0g

Carbohydrates: 16g

Fiber: 4g

Protein: 8g

Cholesterol: 160mg

Oat Bran Muffin

INGREDIENTS

SCALE1x2x3x

¼ cup brown sugar

2 cups Bob Red Mill High Fiber Oat Bran Cereal (if you cannot find at store go to Amazon)

1 cup whole wheat flour

2 tablespoons ground flax meal

2 teaspoons baking powder

2 teaspoons baking soda

½ cup liquid egg whites

1 cup chilled applesauce (no sugar added)

3 tablespoons olive oil

1 ½ cups of frozen cranberries (or any berry you like)

Cook Mode Prevent your screen from going dark

INSTRUCTIONS

Preheat oven to 400 degree

Thoroughly mix brown sugar, oat bran cereal, whole wheat flour, flax meal, baking powder, and baking soda

Add eggs, applesauce, olive oil, and cranberries

Mix with a wooden spoon until well-blended

Spoon into sprayed muffin pans (sprayed with whatever spray oil you use)

Bake at 400 for 15 minutes

Let cool for 10 minutes on a baking rack

NOTES

Oxalate: 4mg   Total Sugar: 6g   Added Sugar: 3g

Yield: 12

NUTRITION

Serving Size: 1

Calories: 145

Sodium: 184mg

Fat: 5g

Saturated Fat: 1g

Unsaturated Fat: 0

Trans Fat: 0

Carbohydrates: 23g

Fiber: 3g

Protein: 4g

Cholesterol: 0

Chicken Meatball and Couscous

INGREDIENTS

SCALE1x2x3x

1/2 red onion, diced

1 beaten egg

2 garlic cloves

1/4 Cup fresh basil

1 Cup of couscous

1 Teaspoon dried oregano

1 Cup cherry tomatoes, halved

1/4 Cup fresh Italian parsely

1/3 Cup bread crumbs

1 pound ground chicken

1 Cup of kale

1/4 cup grated parmesan cheese

1/2 teaspoon paprika

Cook Mode Prevent your screen from going dark

INSTRUCTIONS

Make couscous following directions on package

Dice red onion

Cut tomatoes in half

On medium flame in non-stick pan, saute onion,
when translucent, add tomatoes and kale until soft.

Combine the above veggies with the couscous when everything is done. I also added a TBS of basil and Italian parsley to the above pot.

For the meatballs:

With hands combine ground chicken, beaten egg, garlic bread crumbs, Italian parsley, garlic, basil, parmesan cheese, dried oregano, paprika.

Form in one Tablespoon sized meatballs. Make sure all are consistently sized so they all cook through at the same time.

Bake on a lightly brushed olive oil coated sheet pan for 30 minutes on 400.

Chili Mac

INGREDIENTS

SCALE1x2x3x

2 Teaspoon oregano

2 Teaspoon cumin

1 Tablespoon fresh cilantro

1/4 green pepper

1/4 onion

1 pound ground lean turkey

2 Cups water

1 Tablespoon olive oil

6 ounces of chickpea pasta

2 Tablespoon of non-fat plain greek yogurt

Muir Glenn low sodium diced tomatoes

1/2 cup of frozen corn

Cook Mode Prevent your screen from going dark

INSTRUCTIONS

In a large sauce pot add the olive oil to medium high heat.

Dice up onion and green pepper and add to pot. Add turkey and cook until no pink.

Add diced tomato sauce, water, corn, cumin, oregano, and bring to a boil.

Add pasta to pot and turn down heat to simmer. Pasta will be done in about 8 minutes or according to package instructions. Taste it so it doesn't get too mushy. Chickpea pasta can go from hard to mushy in what seems like a second.

When pasta is done, take off the burner and add greek yoghurt and cilantro.

Oxalate: See Notes Added Sugar: 0g Calcium: 100mg

NUTRITION

Calories: 400

Sugar: 7g

Sodium: 191mg

Fat: 14g

Saturated Fat: 3g

Unsaturated Fat: 9g

Trans Fat: 0g

Carbohydrates: 38g

Fiber: 5g

Protein: 33g

Cholesterol: 84mg

Stoner Mashed Potatoes

COOK TIME: 10 Minutes

TOTAL TIME: 25 minutes

YIELD: 4 Servings 1x

INGREDIENTS

SCALE1x2x3x

2 Tablespoon chives

1/4 Cup of skim milk

1 head cauliflower

1/2 Cup of swiss cheese

2 pats of unsalted butter

Cook Mode Prevent your screen from going dark

INSTRUCTIONS

Preheat oven to 350 degrees

Fill soup pot halfway with water and bring to boil

Break up cauliflower into smaller bits and put in pot when water is boiling

When cauliflower is soft it is done

You can now transfer cauliflower into a food processor or blender. Add the milk (or non dairy milk of your choice), and the butter.

When the mixture is creamy transfer cauliflower into a baking dish. Top with swiss cheese and chives. And cover with aluminum foil. Cook for about 10 minutes or until cheese melts.

NOTES

Oxalate: 0mg Added Sugar: 0mg Calcium: 194mg

NUTRITION

Calories: 121

Sugar: 4g

Sodium: 60mg

Fat: 7g

Saturated Fat: 4g

Unsaturated Fat: 2g

Trans Fat: 0g

Carbohydrates: 8g

Fiber: 3g

Protein: 8g

Cholesterol: 21mg

Low Carb Baby Bella and Broccoli Rice

COOK TIME: 10 Minutes

TOTAL TIME: 25 minutes

YIELD: 2 Servings 1x

INGREDIENTS

SCALE1x2x3x

8 ounces baby bella mushrooms

1 Cup arugula

2 Tablespoon olive oil

1 Tablespoon balsamic vinegar

1 Tablespoon chopped parsley

1/8 Cup of Trader Joe's no-sugar-added cranberries

1 head broccoli

1/2 finely chopped shallot

 bip of black pepper

1/8 Cup of no-salt sunflower seeds

1 garlic clove

sprinkle of parmesan cheese

Cook Mode Prevent your screen from going dark

INSTRUCTIONS

Break the broccoli into florets. Trim the bottom of stems and roughly chop the stems. Put all broccoli and stems into a food processor and pulse a few times until the mixture is the size of rice. You might have to do this in a couple of batches.

In a saute pan, heat one tablespoon of olive oil over medium heat. Add the mushrooms and saute for about 5 minutes or until they start to brown. Stir in the balsamic vinegar and garlic and continue cooking for a few minutes so that the mushrooms are caramelized. Transfer to a bowl when they are done.

Take the other tablespoon of olive oil in the same saute pan over medium high heat. Saute the shallots until they soften- about 4 or so minutes, add the broccoli rice, arugula, and a bit of pepper. Cook the rice stirring frequently for about 3 minutes or until warmed up, but still crisp (don't want broccoli to get mushy).

Fold in the mushroom, parsley, add cranberries, and put some sprinkle some parmesan cheese on top or your favorite (goat, feta, or cheddar). I like the added crunch of no salt sunflower seeds as well.

NOTES

Oxalate: ~30mg Added Sugar: 0g Calcium: 186mg

NUTRITION

Calories: 288

Sugar: 9g

Sodium: 114mg

Fat: 17g

Saturated Fat: 2g

Unsaturated Fat: 12g

Trans Fat: 0g

Carbohydrates: 30g

Fiber: 11g

Protein: 14g

Cholesterol: omg

Low Carb Cauliflower Pizza

COOK TIME: 30 minutes

TOTAL TIME: 45 minutes

YIELD: 2 Servings 1x

INGREDIENTS

SCALE1x2x3x

1 large head cauliflower, grated (about 3 cups), squeezed dry of excess liquid

2 1/2 c. shredded mozzarella, divided

2 large eggs

1 Teaspoon garlic powder

Freshly ground black pepper

3/4 Tomato

1 Tablespoon Italian seasoning

Fresh basil, for garnish

Cook Mode Prevent your screen from going dark

INSTRUCTIONS

STEP 1

Preheat oven to 425° and grease a cast-iron skillet with cooking spray. In a large bowl, combine cauliflower, 1 cup mozzarella, eggs, and garlic powder and season pepper.

STEP 2

Press mixture into skillet, making sure to get up the sides and bake until deeply golden and dry, 25 minutes.

STEP 3

Slice up the fresh tomato and put on top of the crust and sprinkle with the remaining mozzarella.

STEP 4

Sprinkle with basil, slice, and serve.

NOTES

Oxalate: 4mg   Calcium: 524mg   Added Sugar: 0g

NUTRITION

Serving Size: 1/2 Pizza

Calories: 266

Sugar: 2g

Sodium: 537mg

Fat: 18g

Saturated Fat: 8g

Trans Fat: 0g

Carbohydrates: 40

Fiber: 2g

Protein: 23g

Cholesterol: 143mg

Cilantro Lime Vinaigrette

INGREDIENTS

SCALE1x2x3x

1/3 c. chopped fresh cilantro, plus more for garnish

1/4 c. extra-virgin olive oil

Juice of 1 lime

1 tbsp. apple cider vinegar

bip of salt

ground black pepper

1 clove garlic, minced

1/4 tsp. chili powder

Cook Mode Prevent your screen from going dark

INSTRUCTIONS

Pour all ingredients into a blender and mix for 30 to 45 seconds or until thoroughly combined.

Set aside.

Preheat oven to 425°.

NOTES

Oxalate: 0mg

NUTRITION

Calories: 127

Sugar: 0g

Sodium: 38mg

Fat: 14g

Saturated Fat: 2g

Trans Fat: 0g

Carbohydrates: 2g

Fiber: 1g

Protein: 0g

Cholesterol: 0mg

Southwestern Burrito Bowl

PRINT RECIPE

PREP TIME: 10 minutes

COOK TIME: 25 minutes

TOTAL TIME: 35 minutes

YIELD: 4 Servings 1x

INGREDIENTS

SCALE1x2x3x

2 cups sweet potatoes, peeled and cut into 1/2" cubes

1 large red onion, diced

1 tablespoon extra-virgin olive oil

2 c. cooked white rice

1 cup of black beans

1 cup corn (canned or fresh)

1 plum tomato, chopped

1 avocado, sliced

Cook Mode Prevent your screen from going dark

INSTRUCTIONS

Make Cilantro-Lime Vinaigrette: Pour all ingredients into a blender and mix for 30 to 45 seconds or until thoroughly combined. Set aside. Preheat oven to 425°.

On a large baking sheet, place sweet potatoes and onions. Toss with oil and chili powder. Bake 23 to 25 minutes, or until sweet potatoes are tender.

Assemble burrito bowl: Fill each bowl with white rice, black beans, corn, tomato, roasted sweet potato and

onion, and avocado slices. Drizzle with vinaigrette and garnish with extra cilantro and lime, if desired.

NOTES

Oxalate: 25mg   Calcium: 61mg   Added Sugar: 0g

NUTRITION

Calories: 392

Sugar: 8g

Sodium: 136mg

Fat: 12g

Saturated Fat: 2g

Trans Fat: 0g

Carbohydrates: 65g

Fiber: 11g

Protein: 10g

Cholesterol: 0mg